ReNursing Career Consulting

You're A Nurse and Want to Start Your Own Business Workbook

Disclaimer. Although the author and publisher have made every effort to ensure the information provided in this book is correct at press time, they do not assume and hereby disclaim any liability to any party for any loss, damage, or disruption caused by errors or omissions, whether such errors or omissions result from negligence, accident, or any other cause.

This book is not intended as the substitute for the legal advice of attorneys or other law professionals. The reader should regularly consult an attorney or another qualified law professional in matters relating to his/her business and financial matters.

ISBN-13:

978-1547025619

ISBN-10:

1547025611

Printed in the United States of America
10 9 8 7 6 5 4 3 2 1

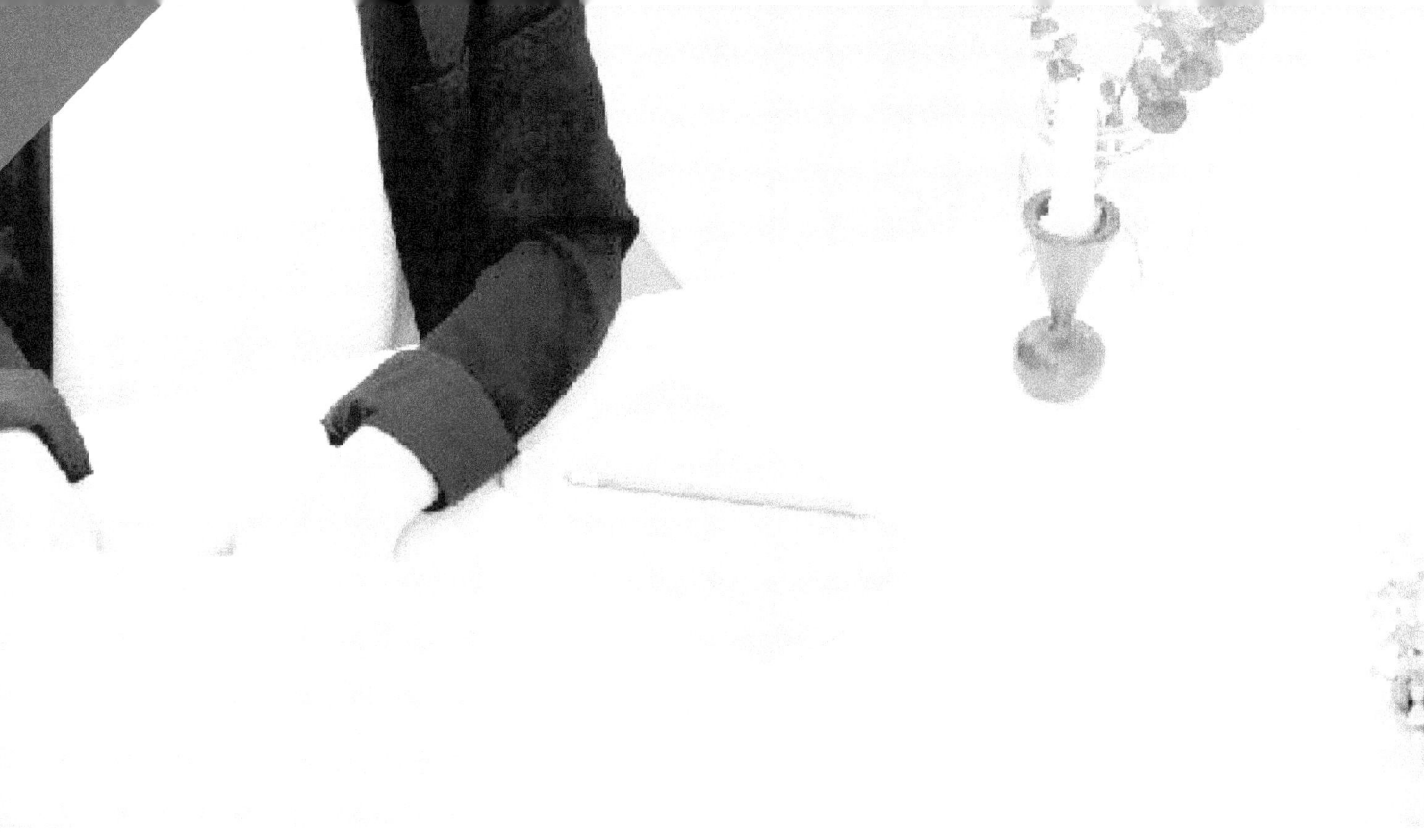

Hi Fellow Nurses!

The choice to work for yourself is clear. Figuring out what type of business you want to start is not. The only thing keeping you from living the life you want to and becoming your own boss is not knowing what you want to offer the world.

Finding your ideal business doesn't have to be a chore. In fact, when you set-up your business to reflect your soul - it won't feel like a chore at all. It will come naturally.

Take me, for instance. The way I talk and carry myself attracts other nurses wanting advice about their careers. I have crafted my business to only attract people who want to work with me.

You need to get really specific on the type of business you want to start. This workbook will take you, step-by-step on just how to accomplish that. Use this workbook to find your business, market it, and scale your empire. Let's start by finding your profitable business idea.

Enjoy!

-Nachole

Find Your Profitable Business Idea

1. Things I'm interested in:

2. Things I'm passionate about:

3. Things I've done and have authority or experience in:

Your business would provide a product or service for your target audience.

Pick 1-2 topics that have the strongest product or service from above. Circle the one you love to start a business on.

Find Your Profitable Business Idea

Copy and pst links to the communities where your target audience hangs out online. A few communities to consider: Facebook groups, Quora, YouTube, Twitter, online forums, etc. Find as many as you can… this step with help your business become profitable!

Community Name	Link

Find Your Profitable Business Idea

Pain	What your business will provide/USP
1. From your list of communities where your audience hangs out, copy and paste your audience's exact complaints, hopes and fears (from comment posts, discussion boards) here. This will help you pinpoint their exact wants and needs.	Think how you can solve the problem VERY SPECIFICALLY targeting the most painful aspect of the problem as possible.
2. EXAMPLE: In the Allnurses forum,	
3	
4	
5	

Find Your Profitable Business Idea

Pain	What your business will provide/USP
6	
7	
8	
9	
10	

Find Your Profitable Business Idea

Use this questionnaire to help profile your audience. Copied from "The Ultimate Sales Letter" by Don Kennedy.

1. What keeps them up at night, indigestion boiling up in their esophagus, eyes, open?

Notes

2. What are they afraid of?

3. What are they angry about? Who are they angry at?

4. What are their top 3 daily frustrations?

5. What trends are occurring and will occur in their business or lives?

Find Your Profitable Business Idea

Use this questionnaire to help profile your audience. Copied from "The Ultimate Sales Letter" by Don Kennedy.

6. What do they secretly, ardently desire the most?

Notes

7. Is there a built-in bias to the way they make decisions? (example: engineers = exceptionally analytical)

8. Do they have their own language?

9. Who else is selling something similar to them, and how?

10. Who else has tried selling them something similar and how has the effort failed?

Are You Suffering From Burnout?

Have you experienced any of these symptoms? You may be suffering from burnout. Take care of yourself!

- [ ] You feel dread or anxiety when you think of going to work

- [ ] You experience sleepless nights wondering if you left something undone, may have harmed a patient, or afraid of disciplinary action from working your last shift?

- [ ] You feel overwhelmed on most days you work

- [ ] You regularly feel like you did not provide good care to your patients because you were so consumed with other things going on at work

- [ ] You find yourself becoming dependent on vices like food, alcohol, or even worse, illegal substances

- [ ] You always feel exhausted and it affects your life outside of work

- [ ] You are always on the lookout for new job opportunities outside of your current job.

- [ ] You are starting not to care about your job performance

List ways you can help alleviate your nursing burnout

_____

_____

_____

_____

The
E.M.P.O.W.E.R
Method

Envision

Dig deep into your soul for these next set of questions

1. What do you dislike about your current job? Is it the pay? The long hours? Working weekends and holidays? Missing your child's events?

Notes

2. What do you like about your job as a nurse? Is it the three shifts per week? The caring aspect of the job

3. Do you still want to used your background as a nurse, just in a different aspect? Or do you want to do something completely different from nursing?

Envision

Dig deep into your soul for these next set of questions

4. If you could choose anything in the world what would be your ideal job?

Notes

5. Where would your like to see yourself in the near future? What about your 5 and 10 year plan?

6. What are your financial goals? An extra $500 per month, $1,000 per month? Or do you want to completely replace your nursing income?

Envison

Make your "Do" and "Don't" list of what you do and don't want to do in your new business

My "Do" List	My "Don't" List

Education

List the forms of education you will use to gain more information
for your new business

Title	Educational Source
Ex: Book	50 + Business Ideas for the Entrepreneurial Nurse

Education

Finding the perfect niche for your business

1. Who is your target audience? Nurses? Doctors?
Patients? The general public?

2. Is your business idea already being done by someone
else? If not, great! That means you already have a niche!

3. If your business idea has already been done, can you
specialize it somehow?

4. What are "extra" services you can offer to your clients that
would carve out a niche for your business?

Plan

Step 1: Snapshot Summary
A snapshot summary is a broad overall coverage of what your business is about and the goals you have for it. Write your business snapshot summary below.

Plan

Use this section to research how others conduct business and how your business will compare.

My Competitor	My Business

Plan

What is your 30 second elevator pitch?

Plan

What will be the general structure of your business, will it be just you or do you need employees? Will it be web-based or brick & mortar?

Plan

What's your marketing plan for your business? Social media, ads, word-of-mouth?

Marketing Strategy	How it will be carried out
Example: Ads	Targeted Amazon and Facebook ads for my products

Plan

What exactly will you provide for your customers and for what price? Are you a service or product-based business?

Service or Product	Price
Example: Books	$2.99- $3.99 for Ebooks and $9.99 for paperback books

Plan

How much money do you need for business start-up costs?

Item	Upfront Cost	Ongoing Cost
Example: Domain name	$9.99	$9.99

Plot Your Own Business Hierarchy

Use this space to draw your own business hierarchy

Organize

Use the template from the "Plan" section to start organizing your business.
Check off each task as it has been finalized.

	Task	Notes
1		
2		
3		
4		
5		

Organize

Use the template from the "Plan" section to start organizing your business. Check off each task as it has been finalized.

	Task	Notes
6		
7		
8		
9		
10		

What's In a Name?

Choosing a name for your business can be fun. Use the guidelines below to choose the best name for your business. List at least 10 potential names for your business

- ☐ The name should not be too long

- ☐ It should give the reader an idea of what your business is about

- ☐ It should be easy to pronounce

- ☐ It should be easy to spell

- ☐ It should be catchy and memorable

- ☐ You will need a similar domain name

Work

Use this space to jot down extra notes for your business.
Example: What do you need for your office set-up? What pages will you
need on your website? What blog topics will you write about?

Work

Use this space to jot down extra notes for your business.
Example: What do you need for your office set-up? What pages will you
need on your website? What blog topics will you write about?

Execute

This section is all about marketing. List your marketing strategies for your business here

	Marketing Strategy	Notes
1	Ex: blogging	High quality blog posts about publishing with good keywords and seo
2		
3		
4		
5		

Execute

This section is all about marketing. List your marketing strategies for your business here

	Marketing Strategy	Notes
6		
7		
8		
9		
10		

Execute

Cold calling: Use this space to write down your cold-calling script. Remember, practice makes perfect, so remember to practice reciting the script out loud before making your calls.

Execute

Cold calling: List the companies you intend to cold call for your business, the contact person and the date you contacted them.

Date	Company	Contact Person
Ex: 5/12	Sole Care Specialists	Mary Jean

Reap

Business Budget. Use this section for your business budget. Additional lines are on the next page. Make as many copies as you need.

Budget Item	Budgeted Amount	Actual Spent	% of Total Budget
Lease/Loan payments			
Utilities			
Phone (cell, fax, landline)			
Accounting fees			
Banking fees			
Insurance (Health, liability, life)			
Legal fees			
Taxes/licenses			
Employee Expenses			
Car (Insurance, loan, maintenance)			
Continuing Education/Training			
Marketing			
Subscriptions			
Office supplies			
Postage/shipping			
P.O. Box			
Website hosting			
Domain name			
Computer software			

Reap

Business Budget. Use this section for your business budget. Make as many copies as you need.

Budget Item	Budgeted Amount	Actual Spent	% of Total Budget

Notes

Use this space for extra notes regarding setting up your business.

Notes

Use this space for extra notes regarding setting up your business.

Notes

Use this space for extra notes regarding setting up your business.

Notes

Use this space for extra notes regarding setting up your business.

Notes

Use this space for extra notes regarding setting up your business.